Harvesting the Spirit Molecule

A Step-by-Step DMT Extraction Handbook

Rogelio L. McCutchen

copyright@2024 Rogelio L. McCutchen all right reserved. No part of this publication should be reproduced in any form or means without a prior written permission form the copyright holder

Introduction 5
   DMT (N,N-Dimethyltryptamine) 5
Chapter One 10
   The Science Behind DMT 10
Chapter Two 19
   Preparation and Safety Guidelines 19
Chapter Three 32
   Methods of DMT Extraction 32
Chapter Four 44
   Purification and Crystallization 44
Chapter Five 58
   Storage and Dosage 58
Chapter Six 71
   The DMT Experience 71
Chapter Seven 87
   Exploring the Cultural and Spiritual Context of DMT 87
Conclusion 104

Introduction

DMT (N,N-Dimethyltryptamine)

DMT, or **N,N-Dimethyltryptamine**, is a powerful psychoactive compound known for its ability to induce profound, immersive experiences that many describe as life-altering. Often referred to as the **"spirit molecule"**, DMT has been revered across cultures, particularly in indigenous South American shamanic practices, where it is a key component in the brew **ayahuasca**. Despite its naturally brief duration, the effects of a DMT experience can be intensely vivid, often producing mystical or otherworldly visions, deep introspective journeys, and encounters with seemingly intelligent entities.

In modern times, DMT has gained attention within both scientific and spiritual communities for its potential to unlock new realms of consciousness and provide a sense of connectedness or oneness with the universe. This book seeks to serve as a comprehensive, step-by-step guide for those interested in responsibly harvesting and extracting DMT from its natural plant sources.

Legal and Ethical Considerations

Before delving into the extraction process, it's essential to understand the legal and ethical boundaries surrounding DMT. DMT is classified as a **Schedule I controlled substance** in many countries, including the United States, making its possession, distribution, and manufacture illegal. However, there are certain religious and cultural contexts, such as the use of ayahuasca in indigenous ceremonies, where DMT is legally protected.

This handbook does not encourage illegal activity; rather, it aims to provide educational insight into the processes involved in extracting DMT, with the intention of promoting safety and harm reduction for those who choose to pursue this knowledge in accordance with their local laws.

Ethical Considerations: Beyond legality, the ethical implications of working with DMT should not be overlooked. DMT is often considered a sacred substance, deeply tied to spiritual practices. Respecting its cultural origins and using it with mindfulness and intention is vital. This book emphasizes the importance of reverence for the plant sources of DMT, sustainable harvesting, and using the molecule in a manner that aligns with both personal integrity and spiritual respect.

Purpose of the Handbook

"Harvesting the Spirit Molecule" is designed to guide readers through the intricate process of DMT extraction, from understanding the basic chemistry behind the molecule to safely executing the extraction procedure. Alongside detailed, step-by-step instructions, this book provides practical advice on dosage, storage, and responsible use, as well as suggestions on how to navigate and integrate the profound experiences that DMT offers.

Throughout this journey, safety will be paramount. Handling chemicals, understanding dosages, and preparing for the psychological intensity of a DMT experience all require careful attention. Whether you are a curious explorer, a spiritual seeker, or someone with an interest in plant-based entheogens, this handbook serves as both a practical and philosophical guide to responsibly engaging with the spirit molecule.

Chapter One

The Science Behind DMT

The Chemistry of DMT

At its core, **N,N-Dimethyltryptamine (DMT)** is a tryptamine alkaloid, a compound closely related to serotonin, melatonin, and other naturally occurring neurotransmitters in the brain. Structurally, DMT consists of an indole ring, a fundamental component shared with many biologically active molecules, and two methyl groups attached to a nitrogen atom (hence the "dimethyl" in its name).

DMT's psychedelic effects are believed to stem from its interaction with **serotonin receptors**, specifically the **5-HT2A receptor** in the brain. This receptor is implicated in mood regulation, perception, and cognition, and its activation by DMT induces the vivid, altered states of consciousness characteristic of the DMT experience. These states are often described as highly visual and deeply introspective, with users experiencing geometric patterns, fractal landscapes, and encounters with "entities."

One of DMT's most fascinating aspects is its presence in both the plant and animal kingdoms. It is endogenous to the human body, produced in small quantities, though the full extent of its physiological role remains a subject of ongoing research. Some theories suggest that DMT may be produced in the **pineal gland**, an area of the brain traditionally linked to spirituality and mysticism, although this claim is still debated.

DMT in Nature

DMT occurs naturally in a wide variety of plants and some animals. These natural sources can be found across diverse ecosystems, from the rainforests of South America to the deserts of the Middle East. Among the most well-known plant sources are species like **Mimosa hostilis**, **Acacia confusa**, and **Psychotria viridis**, many of which have been used for centuries in traditional spiritual practices.

- **Mimosa hostilis (Jurema)**: One of the most common sources used in modern extraction techniques. The root bark contains high concentrations of DMT, making it a popular choice for DIY extractors.

- **Psychotria viridis**: Commonly used in the Amazonian brew **ayahuasca**, where it is combined with **Banisteriopsis caapi**, a vine that contains monoamine oxidase inhibitors (MAOIs), allowing the DMT to be orally active.

- **Acacia species**: Numerous species of the **Acacia** genus contain DMT, including **Acacia confusa** and **Acacia acuminata**, which are gaining popularity for extraction.

Geographic Distribution of DMT-Containing Plants:

- **South America**: Home to the famous **Mimosa hostilis** and

Psychotria viridis, which are central to ayahuasca traditions.
- **Africa**: Some African acacias contain DMT, although they are less frequently utilized in extraction.
- **Australia**: Known for species like **Acacia acuminata**, part of Aboriginal use in traditional spiritual practices.

DMT and the Human Experience

DMT is often referred to as a **"consciousness-expanding"** substance, and its effects are distinct compared to other psychedelics. While molecules like psilocybin and LSD can produce long-lasting, gradual experiences, DMT's effects are **rapid and intense**, usually peaking within minutes of administration and resolving within 15-30 minutes. This unique aspect has earned DMT the nickname of the "businessman's trip," as it delivers profound, immersive experiences in a short window of time.

Interestingly, DMT is thought to be produced naturally in the human body, possibly playing a role in **dreams, near-death experiences, and mystical states**. However, this theory remains speculative, with more research needed to clarify its physiological significance. There's also emerging interest in the possibility that DMT could be involved in **altered states of consciousness** associated with meditation and deep spiritual practice.

Modern Research and Potential Applications

In recent years, research into DMT has gained momentum, particularly as psychedelics re-enter the scientific mainstream for their potential therapeutic benefits. Though much of this research is still in its early stages, there is evidence suggesting that DMT may have applications in treating **mental health conditions** such as **depression, PTSD, and anxiety**. Its ability to induce profound introspective and spiritual experiences is also being explored as a potential tool for **psychotherapy**, especially in contexts where people seek to resolve deep-seated trauma or find meaning in life-altering events.

Several **clinical trials** are underway to better understand DMT's mechanisms, safety profile, and potential therapeutic uses. Some studies have begun exploring the use of DMT in controlled environments as a catalyst for **transformative mental health interventions**, given its ability to provide deep, often life-changing insights in a brief session.

The Pineal Gland and the Mystical Connection

One of the most fascinating and controversial theories surrounding DMT is its potential connection to the **pineal gland**, a small, pine-cone-shaped structure in the brain historically associated with spiritual and mystical experiences. The pineal gland has long been regarded by some spiritual traditions as the "third eye," a conduit for transcendent experiences. Some researchers have speculated that the pineal gland could produce DMT during extraordinary states, such as **birth, death, and near-death experiences**, though this remains unproven.

Regardless of whether the pineal gland is directly involved in DMT production, the compound's capacity to evoke deep spiritual experiences has made it the focus of much interest from both scientific and mystical perspectives. The **"spirit molecule"** thus serves as a bridge between **modern science** and **ancient spiritual practices**, offering insights into the nature of consciousness, reality, and the human experience.

Chapter Two

Preparation and Safety Guidelines

Equipment and Supplies

Before embarking on the process of DMT extraction, having the right tools and materials is critical for both efficiency and safety. Many of the substances involved in extraction, such as solvents and acids, can be hazardous if mishandled. The following checklist includes both essential equipment and suggested optional tools for a smooth and safe extraction process.

Essential Tools and Materials:

- **Plant Material**: Choose a high DMT-yielding plant like **Mimosa**

hostilis root bark or **Acacia confusa**.
- **Glass Containers**: Mason jars or similar glass containers for mixing solutions.
- **Funnels and Filters**: For straining and separating plant material and solvents.
- **Stainless Steel or Glass Stirring Rods**: For safe stirring and mixing.
- **Measuring Scales**: Accurate scales for measuring precise amounts of plant material and chemicals.
- **pH Strips**: To test the acidity or alkalinity of solutions during extraction.
- **Chemicals/Solvents**:
  - **Lye (Sodium Hydroxide)**: Used for the basification step.

- **Naphtha or Heptane**: Solvents used to pull DMT from the basified solution.
- **Distilled Water**: Essential for creating pure, clean solutions.
- **Eye Droppers or Pipettes**: For carefully transferring small amounts of liquid during extraction.
- **Freezer**: Needed for the crystallization of DMT.

Optional Tools:

- **Magnetic Stirrer**: Helps ensure thorough mixing of solutions, particularly useful for large batches.
- **Vacuum Filtration System**: A more efficient way to filter plant material and chemicals, though not strictly necessary.

- **Crystallization Dish**: A glass or Pyrex dish for collecting DMT crystals during the freezing process.
- **Latex or Nitrile Gloves**: To protect your skin from chemicals.

Safety Gear and Environment

Extracting DMT involves working with chemicals that can be corrosive, flammable, or otherwise hazardous. To minimize risk, wearing the appropriate safety gear and maintaining a controlled work environment is essential.

Personal Protective Equipment (PPE):

- **Gloves**: Always wear chemical-resistant gloves (latex or nitrile) to avoid skin contact with lye and solvents.

- **Safety Goggles**: Protect your eyes from splashes of solvents or lye.
- **Respirator Mask**: When working with volatile solvents like naphtha or heptane, a respirator can protect your lungs from inhaling harmful fumes.
- **Long-Sleeved Clothing**: Protect your skin from potential splashes with long sleeves and closed shoes.

Work Environment:

- **Well-Ventilated Area**: Ensure proper airflow to avoid the buildup of toxic fumes. Working outdoors or in a room with an exhaust fan is ideal.

- **No Open Flames**: Many solvents used in DMT extraction are flammable, so avoid working near open flames, sparks, or hot surfaces.
- **Access to Water and Fire Extinguishers**: Keep water on hand for rinsing chemical splashes and have a fire extinguisher available in case of accidental ignition.

Disposal of Chemicals:

- Never pour solvents or chemicals down the drain. Check local regulations for proper chemical disposal, or take them to a hazardous waste facility to ensure safe disposal. Being mindful of environmental responsibility is a key part of ethical extraction.

Precautions and Harm Reduction

Even with proper safety equipment, the process of extracting DMT demands a responsible approach to mitigate risks. Following best practices during extraction, storage, and consumption can protect both the individual and their surroundings.

Chemical Safety:

- **Lye (Sodium Hydroxide)**: Extremely caustic and can cause burns upon contact with skin or eyes. Always handle with care, and mix it slowly into water to avoid dangerous reactions.

- **Solvent Handling**: Solvents like naphtha and heptane are highly volatile and flammable. Always cap containers tightly when not in use, and avoid breathing in fumes. A respirator or working in an outdoor setting is strongly advised.

Dosage and Consumption Safety:

- **Accurate Dosage**: When consuming DMT, whether through smoking or other means, accurate dosing is critical to avoid overwhelming experiences. Beginners should start with a **threshold dose** (approximately 10-15 mg) before advancing to higher doses (20-30 mg for a typical breakthrough).
- **Psychological Readiness**: DMT can induce highly intense and sometimes overwhelming experiences. It's crucial to be mentally and emotionally prepared

before use. Understanding the power of the substance and having a trusted guide or sitter nearby can help facilitate a safe and meaningful experience.

Creating a Safe and Controlled Environment

The setting in which DMT is both extracted and consumed plays a significant role in ensuring safety. A clean, organized workspace is essential for the extraction process, and a peaceful, comfortable environment is key to having a positive DMT experience.

Extraction Environment:

- **Clean and Organized Workspace**: Clear clutter to ensure no cross-contamination of chemicals, and make sure tools are clean and ready for use.

- **Away from Pets and Children**: Ensure that your workspace is inaccessible to pets or children to prevent accidents.

Consumption Environment:

- **Set and Setting**: As with any powerful psychoactive, the mental state ("set") and physical environment ("setting") are critical for a safe and enriching DMT experience. Ensure that the space is quiet, free of distractions, and comfortable, with any potentially harmful objects removed from the area.

- **Trusted Sitter**: Particularly for beginners, having a **trusted sitter**—someone sober who can monitor you during the experience—is a key safety precaution. This individual should be someone you trust deeply and who understands the nature of DMT trips, prepared to provide reassurance if needed.

Responsible Use of DMT

While this handbook provides step-by-step instructions for DMT extraction, it's equally important to emphasize **responsible use** of the substance. As a powerful psychedelic, DMT can trigger profound shifts in consciousness, which some find spiritually rewarding while others may find overwhelming.

Key Principles of Responsible Use:

- **Respect for the Substance:** DMT is often viewed as a sacred molecule. Using it with the proper mindset, intention, and respect helps ensure a more meaningful experience.
- **Intentionality:** Before consuming DMT, it's helpful to set an intention. Whether you're seeking personal insight, healing, or simply exploring consciousness, having a clear intention can shape the outcome of the experience.
- **Frequency:** DMT can be an intense and life-changing experience, and it's important not to overuse it. Taking time between sessions allows for better integration and reflection

on insights gained during the experience.

Risk of Psychological Harm:

- While physical risks of DMT are minimal when used in proper doses, the intensity of its effects can lead to **challenging psychological experiences**. People with a history of mental illness, especially psychosis, should avoid using DMT or any strong psychedelics without medical supervision.

Chapter Three

Methods of DMT Extraction

In this chapter, we explore the various methods for extracting DMT from plant sources. While there are multiple approaches to extraction, this guide focuses on two of the most commonly used techniques: **acid-base extraction** and **straight-to-base (STB) extraction**. Both methods have been successfully used to isolate DMT from plant materials like **Mimosa hostilis** root bark and **Acacia confusa**, yielding high-quality DMT crystals.

Extraction Methods

Basic Principles of Extraction: At the core of any DMT extraction process is the goal of separating DMT from the plant material in which it naturally occurs. This involves breaking down plant fibers, converting the DMT into a form that can be extracted with a solvent, and then crystallizing it for use.

- **Acid-Base Extraction**: This method uses an acidic solution to break down plant matter and extract the DMT, followed by a basification step to release DMT into a solvent. It is highly efficient and produces very pure crystals.
- **Straight-to-Base (STB) Extraction**: A simpler method that skips the acidification step, going straight to a base solution to pull the DMT from the plant material. While

quicker, it may not produce crystals as pure as the acid-base method.

Acid-Base Extraction Method (Detailed Step-by-Step)

The **Acid-Base (A/B) Extraction** method is one of the most effective ways to extract DMT. It involves converting the DMT into a soluble salt form using an acidic solution, and then freeing it as a freebase form through a basification process, allowing it to be extracted with a non-polar solvent.

Step 1: Plant Material Preparation

- **Materials Needed:**
- **DMT-containing plant material** (e.g., Mimosa hostilis root bark)
- Distilled water
- Vinegar (Acetic Acid)

- **Instructions**:
- Measure and grind the plant material into a fine powder to increase the surface area.
- Place the powdered plant material into a large glass container.
- Add a mixture of **distilled water and vinegar** (or another acid) to the container. The acidic solution helps to break down plant fibers and convert DMT into its salt form.
- Let the mixture sit for a few hours, stirring occasionally to ensure even exposure.

Step 2: Acidification Process

- **Materials Needed**:
- Distilled water
- pH strips
- **Instructions**:

- Check the pH of the acidic solution using pH strips. The ideal pH for this step is between **3 and 4**.
- If the pH is too high, add more acid (e.g., vinegar) to lower the pH. If it is too low, add more water to balance it out.
- Let the plant material soak in the acidic solution for a few hours to ensure full extraction of the DMT salt.

Step 3: Basification and DMT Release

1. **Materials Needed**:
- Lye (sodium hydroxide)
- Distilled water
- Protective gloves and goggles
2. **Instructions**:

- In a separate container, dissolve **lye** (sodium hydroxide) in water to create a **basic solution** (pH > 12). Always add lye to water, not water to lye, to avoid a dangerous reaction.
- Slowly add the basic solution to the acidic plant mixture. The basification process converts the DMT salt into a freebase form, which is insoluble in water but soluble in non-polar solvents.
- Stir gently but thoroughly to ensure the solution is fully mixed. The mixture will turn black or dark brown as the base reacts with the plant material.

Step 4: Solvent Extraction

1. **Materials Needed**:

- Non-polar solvent (e.g., naphtha or heptane)
- Pipette or eye dropper

2. **Instructions**:
- Add a small amount of non-polar solvent to the basified solution. This solvent will pull the DMT freebase from the solution into itself.
- Stir the mixture gently and let it sit for about 30 minutes to allow the DMT to dissolve into the solvent.
- Carefully use a pipette to separate the top solvent layer (containing DMT) from the rest of the solution. Avoid pulling up the dark liquid beneath the solvent layer.

Step 5: Crystallization

1. **Materials Needed**:
- Freezer

- Glass dish

2. **Instructions**:
- Place the solvent (now containing dissolved DMT) in a glass dish.
- Put the dish in a freezer for 24 to 48 hours. Over time, DMT crystals will begin to form as the solvent cools.
- Once the crystals have fully precipitated, carefully pour off the remaining solvent, leaving behind pure DMT crystals.
- Let the crystals dry completely before use.

STB (Straight-to-Base) Extraction Method (Simplified Step-by-Step)

The **Straight-to-Base (STB)** method skips the initial acidification step, going straight into basification and solvent extraction. While easier and faster, the

STB method can sometimes result in slightly less pure DMT crystals due to impurities not being neutralized by the acid step.

Step 1: Plant Material Preparation

- Grind the **Mimosa hostilis root bark** or **Acacia confusa** into a fine powder.
- Place the powder into a large glass container.

Step 2: Basification

1. **Materials Needed**:
- Lye (sodium hydroxide)
- Distilled water
2. **Instructions**:
- Prepare a **lye-water solution** by slowly adding lye to water. Ensure the solution is fully dissolved.

- Pour the lye solution into the container with the plant material. Stir thoroughly to ensure that the plant material is fully submerged and reacting with the base.

Step 3: Solvent Extraction

1. **Materials Needed**:
- Non-polar solvent (e.g., naphtha or heptane)
2. **Instructions**:
- Add non-polar solvent to the basified mixture.
- Stir and let the solution sit for 30 minutes to an hour. The DMT will dissolve into the solvent layer, which will float on top.
- Use a pipette to carefully extract the solvent layer from the dark base solution below.

Step 4: Crystallization

- Place the solvent in a glass dish and freeze it for 24 to 48 hours to precipitate DMT crystals.
- Pour off the solvent and allow the crystals to dry before use.

Comparison of Acid-Base vs. STB Methods

Acid-Base Method:

- **Pros**: Produces highly pure DMT crystals; ideal for those seeking the highest quality product.
- **Cons**: Requires more steps, equipment, and time.

STB Method:

- **Pros**: Simplified, faster process; requires fewer materials.

- **Cons**: May yield slightly less pure DMT crystals.

Both methods are effective and commonly used in the DMT extraction community, but the choice of method often comes down to a balance between time, convenience, and desired purity of the final product.

Chapter Four

Purification and Crystallization

Once DMT has been extracted using either the **Acid-Base** or **Straight-to-Base (STB)** method, the next crucial step is to **purify** the compound and maximize its crystallization quality. Purification ensures that any residual plant matter, solvents, or impurities are removed, leaving behind high-purity DMT crystals ready for use.

This chapter covers essential purification techniques, tips for optimizing crystallization, and troubleshooting common issues encountered during the crystallization process.

Why Purification Is Important

DMT extracted from plant material can contain impurities such as plant oils, fats, and trace chemicals from solvents or lye. Impurities can affect both the **potency** and **experience** of DMT. Purification ensures:

- **Cleaner, smoother consumption**: Especially important when smoking or vaporizing DMT.
- **Maximized potency**: Removal of impurities ensures you're consuming only DMT, with no inert or harmful substances.
- **Better crystallization**: Pure DMT forms larger, more defined crystals, which are more aesthetically pleasing and easier to handle.

Recrystallization Process

The most common purification technique for DMT is **recrystallization**, which involves dissolving the DMT in a solvent, filtering out impurities, and then recrystallizing the purified DMT from the solvent.

Step-by-Step Recrystallization Process:

Step 1: Dissolving the DMT

1. **Materials Needed**:
- DMT crystals from extraction
- Clean, high-quality **non-polar solvent** (e.g., naphtha or heptane)
- Heat source (optional)
2. **Instructions**:

- Take the extracted DMT crystals and place them into a clean glass container.
- Add just enough warm **naphtha** or **heptane** to dissolve the DMT. If the DMT does not dissolve easily at room temperature, gently heat the solvent in a hot water bath (do not use direct flame or excessive heat due to the flammability of solvents).
- Stir the mixture gently until all the DMT dissolves into the solvent. The solution should be clear and free of solid particles.

Step 2: Removing Impurities

1. **Materials Needed**:
- Fine mesh filter or coffee filter
- Glass funnel
2. **Instructions**:

- Once the DMT has fully dissolved, you'll likely notice some undissolved particles in the solution. These are impurities must be removed urgently.
- Set up a glass funnel with a **coffee filter** or fine mesh filter and carefully pour the solution through it into another clean glass container. The filter will trap any undissolved impurities.
- If necessary, repeat this step to ensure the solution is completely free of solid debris.

Step 3: Recrystallization

1. **Materials Needed**:
- Freezer
- Crystallization dish
2. **Instructions**:

- After filtering out the impurities, place the filtered solution into a shallow glass dish (Pyrex or similar) to maximize surface area.
- Place the dish in the freezer for 24 to 48 hours. Over time, DMT crystals will begin to precipitate out of the solvent as it cools.
- As the solvent temperature drops, **large, clear DMT crystals** should form on the bottom and sides of the dish.
- After 48 hours, carefully pour off the remaining solvent, leaving the crystallized DMT behind.

Step 4: Drying the Crystals

1. **Instructions**:
- Once the DMT crystals have been separated from the solvent, allow

them to air dry for several hours to ensure all residual solvent evaporates.
- Use a small fan or place the crystals in a cool, dry area to speed up the drying process. Avoid direct heat to prevent melting the crystals.

Freeze Precipitation Method

An alternative and often complementary method to recrystallization is **freeze precipitation**. This technique takes advantage of the fact that DMT becomes insoluble in non-polar solvents at cold temperatures, leading to the formation of crystals.

Step-by-Step Freeze Precipitation Process:

Step 1: Dissolving in Solvent

- Dissolve the extracted DMT in warm naphtha or heptane, similar to the recrystallization process.
- Ensure all DMT is fully dissolved by gently heating the solvent (in a hot water bath, if necessary).

Step 2: Freezing the Solution

- Place the dissolved DMT solution in a shallow glass dish or jar.
- Place the dish in the freezer and leave it undisturbed for **24-48 hours**.

Step 3: Collecting the Crystals

- After 24 to 48 hours, you should see **white crystalline DMT** forming at the bottom and sides of the dish.
- Carefully pour off the solvent, leaving the crystals behind.
- Let the crystals dry completely in a well-ventilated area before use.

Common Purification Issues and Solutions

Issue 1: DMT Doesn't Fully Dissolve in Solvent

- **Cause**: Low solvent temperature or insufficient solvent used.
- **Solution**: Gently warm the solvent (using a hot water bath) and stir to help the DMT fully dissolve. Use just enough solvent to dissolve the

crystals without adding too much excess.

Issue 2: No Crystal Formation in Freezer

- **Cause**: DMT may not have been fully dissolved, or the solvent is too dilute.
- **Solution**: Ensure that the DMT is fully dissolved in the solvent before freezing. If the solution is too dilute, evaporate some of the solvent to increase concentration before attempting freeze precipitation again.

Issue 3: Impure Crystals After Recrystallization

- **Cause**: Insufficient filtering or use of a contaminated solvent.

- **Solution**: Repeat the filtering step to remove more impurities. Make sure to use a clean solvent and avoid cross-contaminating equipment.

Issue 4: Crystals Remain Sticky or Oily

- **Cause**: Residual solvent hasn't fully evaporated.
- **Solution**: Allow more drying time. Place the crystals in front of a fan or in a low-humidity environment to speed up evaporation. Avoid using direct heat, as it can degrade the DMT.

Maximizing Crystal Growth

The size and appearance of DMT crystals can vary, but larger, well-formed crystals are often a sign of good purification and proper handling. Here are some tips to maximize crystal growth:

- **Slow Cooling**: Crystals grow best when the solution cools slowly and uniformly. Avoid rapid cooling, as it may result in smaller, less defined crystals.
- **Shallow Dishes**: Use a shallow crystallization dish to spread out the solvent, allowing for a larger surface area for crystals to form.
- **Patience**: Let the crystals form over a period of 48 hours for best results. Rushing the process can lead to incomplete crystallization and smaller crystals.

Final Steps: Storing Purified DMT Crystals

After purification and crystallization, it's essential to store your DMT crystals properly to maintain their purity and potency.

1. **Storage Tips**:
- Store the DMT in **airtight containers** to prevent exposure to air and moisture, which can degrade the compound over time.
- Keep the container in a **cool, dark place**, away from direct sunlight or heat, as these can accelerate the breakdown of DMT.
- For longer-term storage, consider keeping the DMT in a freezer or other cold environment, ensuring

that it remains stable for months or even years.

Chapter Five

Storage and Dosage

After successfully extracting and purifying DMT, proper storage and responsible dosing are essential to maintaining its **potency**, **safety**, and **effectiveness**. This chapter provides a comprehensive guide on how to store DMT to prevent degradation and how to approach dosing, considering the potency and variability of the DMT experience.

Storage of DMT Crystals

Proper storage is crucial for preserving the **quality** and **effectiveness** of your DMT crystals over time. Exposure to air, moisture, light, or heat can degrade the compound, affecting both its potency and usability.

Best Practices for Storage

- **Airtight Containers**: Use glass or plastic airtight containers to seal off the DMT from environmental factors. Airtight containers prevent air and humidity from reaching the crystals, both of which can degrade the compound.
- **Avoid Light Exposure**: UV rays from sunlight can degrade DMT over time. Store your DMT in a **dark, opaque container**, or keep it in a cool, dark space to avoid exposure to light. Alternatively, wrap the container in aluminum foil for additional protection.

- **Temperature Control**: Heat can accelerate the breakdown of DMT. The ideal storage temperature is **cool or cold**, but room temperature can be acceptable for shorter periods. For longer storage, consider keeping your DMT in a freezer or refrigerator to help preserve its potency for months or even years.
- **Desiccants**: Include small desiccant packets (silica gel) in your container to prevent moisture from entering the storage environment. Humidity can cause your DMT to clump or degrade, particularly in regions with high humidity levels.

Long-Term Storage

- For extended storage (months or longer), a **freezer** is highly recommended. Make sure the container is well-sealed to prevent condensation from forming when taken out of cold storage.

- Ensure the DMT crystals are completely dry before storage, as moisture could freeze and create unwanted residue or degradation.

Signs of Degradation

- **Color Changes**: Freshly extracted and purified DMT crystals are typically **white or light yellow**. If your DMT starts to take on a darker yellow, orange, or brown tint, it may be an indicator of degradation, though it may still be effective.
- **Texture Changes**: DMT crystals should be solid and dry. If your DMT becomes sticky, oily, or mushy, it

could be due to moisture exposure or breakdown from improper storage conditions.

DMT Dosage

DMT is one of the most potent psychoactive compounds, and **accurate dosing** is essential for both safety and the experience itself. The dosage level can dramatically affect the **intensity**, **duration**, and **nature** of the DMT experience.

Factors Affecting Dosage

The ideal DMT dosage can vary based on several factors, including:

- **Experience Level**: Beginners may want to start with lower doses, while more experienced users might be comfortable with higher doses.

- **Mode of Administration**: The method of consumption (e.g., vaporizing, smoking, oral administration with an MAOI) affects how much DMT is absorbed and how intense the experience will be.
- **Body Chemistry**: Individual metabolism and tolerance can influence how the body responds to a specific dose of DMT.
- **Setting**: The mental and physical environment in which DMT is used (commonly referred to as "set and setting") plays a significant role in the experience.

Typical DMT Dosages

For the most common method of administration—**vaporizing or smoking DMT freebase**—dosage guidelines are as follows:

- **Threshold Dose (Light)**: 5-10 mg
Effects: Mild, subtle visual and sensory alterations. Good for beginners to gauge sensitivity.
- **Low Dose**: 10-20 mg
Effects: Moderate visual and auditory distortions. A good introduction to the DMT experience without fully immersive effects.
- **Common Dose (Breakthrough Threshold)**: 20-30 mg
Effects: Intense visuals, with full immersion in the DMT experience. Possible **breakthrough** into another realm or dimension. This dose level

is considered powerful for most users.

- **High Dose**: 30-50 mg+ Effects: Profound, often overwhelming visuals and experiences, complete loss of connection with physical reality. This dose is reserved for experienced users seeking a complete and extended breakthrough.

Administration Methods

- **Vaporizing or Smoking**: The most common way to consume DMT freebase is by vaporizing it in a glass pipe or using a vaporizer. This method provides a rapid onset, often within **seconds to minutes**, and a peak experience lasting 5-15 minutes. Effects can last up to **30 minutes** with a gradual comedown.

- **Changa**: A smokable blend of DMT-infused herbs, such as **Caapi** leaves. Changa extends the duration of the DMT experience and provides a gentler onset and longer trip duration, generally **20-40 minutes**. Dosage with changa depends on the DMT concentration in the blend.
- **Oral Consumption (Ayahuasca)**: When combined with a **MAOI** (Monoamine Oxidase Inhibitor), such as **Banisteriopsis caapi** or **harmaline**, DMT can be taken orally in a brew like **Ayahuasca**. This route results in a significantly longer experience, typically **4-6 hours**, with a more gradual onset and less intense peak, though the journey is

often deeper. Dosage depends heavily on the specific MAOI and DMT concentrations in the brew.

Measuring Your Dose

To ensure accurate dosing, always use a **milligram scale** when measuring out DMT crystals. Given the compound's potency, small differences in dose can lead to significantly different experiences.

- **Microdosing**: For sub-threshold effects, a very small dose (1-5 mg) can be used. Microdosing is for users looking for minimal psychoactive effects and more subtle mental or spiritual clarity.
- **Measuring for Breakthrough**: For those seeking a **breakthrough** dose, starting with **20-25 mg** is

typically recommended for an intense but manageable experience. Work your way up gradually if more intensity is desired.

Responsible Use and Safety Considerations

DMT is an extremely powerful and fast-acting psychedelic. It is essential to approach dosing with care and responsibility.

Set and Setting

- **Set**: Your **mindset** going into the experience is crucial. Be in a positive, open, and calm state of mind to avoid negative or overwhelming experiences.
- **Setting**: A safe, comfortable, and quiet environment is ideal for using

DMT. Since the effects come on rapidly, ensure that you are in a space where you feel secure and are unlikely to be disturbed.

Presence of a Sitter

Having a **sober sitter** is highly recommended, especially for high-dose experiences. The sitter can offer support, ensure your physical safety, and provide reassurance during or after the experience.

Dosage Titration

If you are new to DMT or unsure of your personal tolerance, **titrate your dose**. Start with a lower amount and gradually increase until you find your ideal dosage. This minimizes the risk of overwhelming or negative experiences.

Health Considerations

- DMT is generally safe in terms of physiological effects, but individuals with **heart conditions** or **severe psychological disorders** should avoid it due to its intense effects on the nervous system.
- If using oral DMT in combination with a **MAOI** (Ayahuasca), be aware of potential **dietary and drug interactions**. MAOIs inhibit the breakdown of DMT and other substances in the body, meaning certain foods and medications (like antidepressants) can cause adverse reactions.

Chapter Six

The DMT Experience

The **DMT experience** is often described as one of the most profound, transformative, and intense psychedelic journeys available. This chapter delves into the nature of DMT experiences, providing an understanding of the common stages, sensory perceptions, and mental and emotional landscapes that are often encountered. Whether you're approaching DMT for the first time or deepening an existing relationship with the substance, this chapter offers insights into what you may encounter during the journey.

The Phases of a DMT Trip

DMT experiences generally unfold in **distinct phases** that occur rapidly, often within seconds of inhalation or administration. These phases can vary in intensity based on the dose and the individual's mental state, but they generally follow a recognizable pattern.

Onset (0-30 seconds)

- The DMT experience begins **almost immediately** after smoking or vaporizing, with effects often felt within 10-30 seconds. The onset is rapid and can be overwhelming, as users are suddenly transported into a highly altered state of consciousness.
- **Physical Sensations**: Users often report a feeling of pressure or

energy, which can feel as if the body is being pulled or pushed. This sensation is typically short-lived but intense.

- **Visual Distortions**: During the onset, bright geometric patterns and fractal imagery begin to form, usually with eyes closed but sometimes with eyes open. Colors may become unusually vibrant, and everything may seem to pulse or ripple.
- **Loss of Ego**: The sense of **self** or personal identity may begin to dissolve quickly, leaving users feeling as if they are no longer in control of their own body or mind. This is often described as a **disassociation** from the ego.

Peak (1-5 minutes)

- The peak of the DMT experience is often referred to as the **breakthrough phase**, where users may feel like they are transported to another realm or dimension. This phase is marked by:
- **Immersion in Visuals**: Complex, fast-moving visuals of intense color and light. Users often describe intricate geometries, tunnels, or landscapes that seem to be alive or sentient.
- **Presence of Entities**: Many users report encountering **beings** or **entities** during the peak of the experience. These entities vary widely, from alien-like figures to ethereal presences or even familiar forms. Encounters with these

entities are often highly emotional, with feelings ranging from awe and wonder to fear or love.

- **Loss of Time and Space**: The normal sense of time and spatial awareness dissolves. Users often feel they've entered a place outside of time, where moments can feel eternal or fleeting.
- **Spiritual or Mystical Experience**: DMT's peak is often described as deeply spiritual. Users may feel as though they've encountered the divine, accessed higher levels of consciousness, or entered a sacred space. Many describe this as a **oneness with the universe** or a profound understanding of life, death, and existence.

Comedown (5-15 minutes)

- After the peak, the experience gradually begins to taper off. This **comedown** period allows users to start returning to baseline reality, though visuals may persist.
- **Integration of Experience**: During the comedown, the mind often tries to make sense of what occurred during the peak. Memories of the encounter, the entities, or any messages or insights gained during the trip start to resurface and may feel clearer.
- **Visual Echoes**: While the intensity of the visuals fades, echoes of geometric shapes, patterns, or color shifts may persist for a short time after the peak has passed.
- **Emotional Processing**: Emotions may feel raw or heightened during

the comedown. Some users describe feelings of immense **peace**, **love**, or **gratitude**, while others may feel overwhelmed or confused by the magnitude of what they experienced.

Aftereffects (15-30 minutes)

- By the 15-30 minute mark, users typically return to their normal state of consciousness. However, lingering aftereffects, such as feelings of awe, introspection, or clarity, may persist for hours or even days after the experience.
- **Emotional Reflection**: Many users find themselves reflecting deeply on their experience, often leading to a period of introspection or personal growth.

- **Enhanced Sensory Perception**: Even after the primary effects have worn off, some users report heightened sensitivity to light, sound, or other sensory stimuli for a short period.

Visuals and Sensory Alterations

DMT is famous for its overwhelming visual effects, but the **sensory experience** extends beyond just sight. The combination of visual, auditory, and sometimes tactile alterations creates a complete immersion into the experience.

Visuals

- **Geometric Patterns**: DMT produces some of the most vivid and complex visuals of any psychedelic.

Fractals, **grids**, and **mosaic-like shapes** move and evolve, often with intricate detail and rich color.

- **Dimensional Shifts**: Many users report the sense of traveling through multiple layers of reality or through portals and tunnels that appear to lead to different worlds or dimensions.

- **Hyper-Realism**: The visual experience often feels more real than reality itself, with an incredible sharpness and vibrancy to the images that emerge.

Auditory Alterations

- **Internal Sounds**: Users frequently report hearing **internal sounds**, such as buzzing, humming, or mechanical noises, especially during

the onset of the experience. Some describe these sounds as guiding the trip or leading to the breakthrough.
- **Music and Tones**: For some, the experience may include celestial or otherworldly music, or it can make ordinary sounds (music, voices, environmental sounds) feel more significant or sacred.

Tactile Sensations

- **Body Dissociation**: Many users report feeling disconnected from their physical body, often to the point of being unaware of their body's presence.
- **Energy Flows**: Some people experience waves of energy or vibrations flowing through their

body, often concentrated in the head, chest, or spine.

Encounters with Entities

One of the most well-known and often-discussed aspects of the DMT experience is the **encounter with entities**. These beings appear during the peak of the experience and can range from abstract shapes or energies to fully formed humanoid or alien-like figures.

Types of Entities

- **Machine Elves**: Often described as small, playful, and sentient beings that inhabit the DMT realm. They seem to interact with users, sometimes offering guidance or observing the experience.

- **Alien Beings**: Some users encounter beings that resemble traditional descriptions of extraterrestrial life, including humanoids with large eyes or energy beings that communicate telepathically.
- **Geometric or Abstract Entities**: Not all entities take on familiar shapes. Some appear as complex geometries or fluid shapes that seem to possess consciousness.

Interaction with Entities

- **Communication**: Many users report some form of communication with these beings, though it is often telepathic rather than verbal. The messages can be profound, offering wisdom or insight into personal or universal truths.

- **Guidance or Healing**: Some users feel that the entities are benevolent and offer emotional or spiritual healing, while others may experience them as neutral or indifferent.
- **Emotional Responses**: The encounter with entities can be overwhelming and emotional. Many describe feelings of **awe**, **love**, or **fear**, depending on the nature of the interaction.

Psychological and Emotional States

The DMT experience can evoke a wide range of emotions and psychological states, from the blissful and euphoric to the deeply challenging and overwhelming.

Euphoria and Bliss

- **Feelings of Oneness**: DMT users often report feelings of **unconditional love**, **unity**, and connection with all of existence, leading to profound spiritual or mystical revelations.
- **Transcendence**: Many describe a sensation of transcending their ego, body, and physical limitations, connecting with a higher consciousness or divine presence.

Anxiety and Fear

- **Overwhelm**: For some, the rapid onset and intensity of the experience can trigger feelings of anxiety or fear, especially for first-time users or those who feel unprepared for the journey.

- **Ego Death**: The dissolution of the ego can be frightening for individuals who are not familiar with such experiences. The loss of personal identity or sense of control can lead to challenging moments of existential confrontation.

Insights and Integration

- Many users return from a DMT trip with profound insights into their personal life, relationships, and place in the universe. These insights may take time to integrate and fully understand, but they can lead to lasting changes in perspective and behavior.

Integration: Making Sense of the Experience

The true value of a DMT journey often lies in how the experience is **integrated** into everyday life. The insights, emotions, and revelations from a DMT trip can be life-changing but require careful reflection and application.

Post-Trip Reflection

- **Journaling**: Many users find it helpful to write down their experiences immediately after a DMT trip to capture the emotions, visuals, and insights before they fade.
- **Discussion**: Talking about the experience with trusted friends, a community, or a guide can

Chapter Seven

Exploring the Cultural and Spiritual Context of DMT

DMT has a long history of **cultural, spiritual, and religious significance**, particularly in indigenous traditions across South America. This chapter explores the deep roots of DMT in various spiritual contexts, how it has been used for centuries in ritual and healing practices, and its growing influence in modern psychedelic spirituality.

Historical Use of DMT in Indigenous Cultures

DMT-containing plants have been used for thousands of years by indigenous peoples, primarily in the Amazon basin.

The primary method of consumption in these cultures is through **Ayahuasca**, a brew made from combining DMT-rich plants with an **MAOI** to make the compound orally active. This section delves into the ancient and ongoing traditions surrounding DMT in these communities.

The Role of Ayahuasca in Indigenous Tribes

- **Shamanic Practices**: In tribes such as the **Shipibo-Conibo**, **Asháninka**, and **Yawanawá**, Ayahuasca is central to shamanic traditions. Shamans, or **curanderos**, use the brew for divination, healing, and spiritual exploration. They act as guides during ceremonies, helping participants navigate their visions and spiritual journeys.

- **Ritual and Healing**: Ayahuasca ceremonies are often conducted with a focus on healing, both **physically** and **spiritually**. Shamans believe the brew allows them to communicate with the spirit world and diagnose illnesses, removing negative energies or spiritual blockages from those seeking healing.
- **Visionary States**: The visions experienced during Ayahuasca ceremonies are seen as messages from the spirit world. These visions may provide insights, solutions to problems, or deep emotional healing. Participants often seek Ayahuasca not just for personal

growth but for guidance from the **spirit realm**.

Other Indigenous Uses of DMT-Containing Plants

- **Yopo and Vilca**: Apart from Ayahuasca, some South American indigenous groups use **Yopo** and **Vilca**, which are snuffs made from DMT-containing seeds of plants like **Anadenanthera peregrina**. These snuffs are typically inhaled during rituals to induce visionary states, connect with the spirit world, or gain wisdom from ancestral spirits.
- **Jurema**: In northeastern Brazil, the root bark of the **Jurema** plant (Mimosa tenuiflora) contains DMT and is used in spiritual ceremonies, especially in **Afro-Brazilian**

religions like **Umbanda** and **Jurema cults**. Jurema is used in rituals to facilitate communication with spirits and is an essential tool for **mystical journeys**.

DMT in Modern Spirituality and Psychedelic Culture

In recent decades, DMT has gained popularity in **Western cultures**, where it is often used for **spiritual awakening**, **consciousness exploration**, and **personal transformation**. This section explores the evolution of DMT's role in modern spirituality and the psychedelic movement.

The Psychedelic Renaissance

- **Revival of Interest**: The late 20th century saw a resurgence in the use of psychedelics for spiritual and psychological exploration. Researchers like **Dr. Rick Strassman** pioneered clinical studies on DMT, sparking a renewed interest in its potential for **consciousness expansion** and **mystical experiences**. Strassman's work, particularly his book *DMT: The Spirit Molecule*, was pivotal in shifting the perception of DMT in Western contexts, associating it with **spiritual awakening** and **entheogenic** experiences.
- **Psychedelic Communities**: DMT has become a central component of modern psychedelic culture, with

users exploring it for both recreational and spiritual purposes. Psychedelic communities around the world host **DMT retreats**, **Ayahuasca ceremonies**, and other forms of ritual use that draw from indigenous traditions while adapting to contemporary spiritual practices.

DMT and the Search for Higher Consciousness

- **Mystical and Transcendent States**: Many modern users approach DMT with the goal of achieving **mystical experiences**. The rapid onset and intensity of DMT often lead to profound feelings of unity with the universe, connection with the divine, and a **sense of timelessness** or **infinity**. These experiences are often described as **ego dissolution**, where the individual self merges into a greater cosmic whole.

- **Consciousness Exploration**: For many, DMT is not just a tool for spiritual awakening but a **gateway** to exploring the boundaries of human consciousness. The vivid, often alien landscapes encountered during DMT trips suggest the existence of other dimensions or realms of consciousness, leading users to contemplate the nature of reality, life after death, and the potential for multi-dimensional experiences.

Spiritual Interpretations of DMT Experiences

Many DMT users, both past and present, interpret their experiences through a **spiritual lens**. The overwhelming sense of connection, unity, and the presence of entities often leads to religious or spiritual interpretations of DMT encounters.

Encounters with Divine or Cosmic Beings

- **God or Higher Power**: Some users interpret their experience as a direct encounter with **God**, a **universal consciousness**, or a **cosmic intelligence**. These experiences often leave participants with a profound sense of purpose or understanding of the divine nature of existence.

- **Angels, Demons, or Spirits**: In some cases, entities encountered during DMT trips are interpreted as **spiritual beings**, ranging from angels and spirit guides to tricksters or demonic presences. These experiences are often deeply emotional and can be transformative, providing guidance or teaching through symbolic visions.

Reincarnation and the Afterlife

- **Past Lives**: Some DMT users report encountering visions of **past lives** or feeling as though they've lived multiple existences. These experiences often provoke deep reflection on the nature of reincarnation and karma.

- **The Afterlife**: Given the intensity of the ego-dissolving effects of DMT, many users describe the experience as akin to **death** and **rebirth**. This has led some to speculate that DMT could provide a glimpse into what happens after death, with users reporting feelings of entering a "**spirit world**" or experiencing a **life review**.

Shamanic Cosmology and Healing

- In shamanic cosmology, the use of DMT-rich Ayahuasca is often viewed as a tool for spiritual and physical healing. The visions and insights gained during the journey are interpreted as messages from the spirit world, meant to heal the soul and guide the user towards a more balanced and harmonious life.

- **Soul Retrieval**: In some indigenous traditions, Ayahuasca is used to perform **soul retrieval**—a process by which shamans reclaim parts of a person's spirit that have been lost due to trauma, illness, or life's difficulties. This healing process is considered essential for restoring emotional and spiritual wholeness.

Ayahuasca Tourism and Ethical Considerations

With the rising interest in Ayahuasca and DMT, many Westerners travel to **South America** to participate in Ayahuasca retreats and ceremonies. While this can be a transformative experience, there are important ethical considerations around **cultural appropriation**, the commodification of indigenous practices, and the impact on local communities.

The Rise of Ayahuasca Tourism

- **Spiritual Seekers**: Each year, thousands of people travel to the Amazon in search of healing and spiritual enlightenment through Ayahuasca ceremonies led by indigenous shamans. These retreats often promise deep psychological healing, spiritual awakening, and connection to ancient wisdom.
- **Commercialization**: The popularity of Ayahuasca has led to a boom in **Ayahuasca tourism**, where ceremonies are often

commercialized, and some shamans may cater to the demands of tourists rather than preserving the authenticity of the tradition.

Ethical Dilemmas

- **Cultural Appropriation**: Critics argue that Ayahuasca tourism can be seen as **cultural appropriation**, where indigenous traditions are exploited for profit without respecting their cultural significance or origins.
- **Exploitation of Indigenous Communities**: The influx of tourism has impacted many indigenous communities, leading to the exploitation of local shamans and disruption of traditional practices. Some shamans are pressured to

cater to tourists rather than maintaining the spiritual integrity of the ceremonies.

Responsible Participation

- For those interested in exploring Ayahuasca or DMT in an authentic and respectful way, it is important to **research** the ethics of participating in such ceremonies. Ensuring that the retreat centers are ethically run, and that shamans are properly compensated and respected, helps to mitigate the negative impact of Ayahuasca tourism.

Integrating Indigenous Wisdom into Modern Practices

As DMT continues to gain popularity in Western contexts, there is a growing movement to **honor the indigenous origins** of these practices while integrating them into modern spiritual frameworks.

Respecting the Source

- Many modern users and facilitators emphasize the importance of acknowledging the indigenous cultures from which Ayahuasca and DMT originate. This includes **paying homage to the spiritual practices**, recognizing the knowledge passed down through generations, and **avoiding the commodification** of these sacred medicines.

Blending Traditions

- Some contemporary practitioners blend **indigenous shamanic wisdom** with other spiritual traditions, creating a **hybrid** form of practice that respects the roots of DMT while adapting it for modern spiritual seekers. This may include combining Ayahuasca with practices like **yoga**, **meditation**, or **energy healing** to create a holistic approach to personal growth.

Conclusion

The exploration of DMT reveals its profound complexity, intertwining science, culture, spirituality, and personal experience. As a powerful entheogen, DMT has been utilized for centuries by indigenous peoples for healing, spiritual guidance, and connection with the divine. In contemporary society, it is increasingly embraced for its potential to expand consciousness, provoke profound insights, and foster personal transformation.

However, the growing interest in DMT and Ayahuasca also raises important ethical considerations, particularly concerning cultural appropriation and the commercialization of indigenous practices. As modern seekers navigate these experiences, it is crucial to approach them with respect and awareness of their historical and cultural significance.

Ultimately, DMT serves as a bridge between the known and the unknown, inviting individuals to explore the depths of their consciousness, confront existential questions, and cultivate a deeper understanding of their place within the universe. As research and interest in psychedelics continue to evolve, the insights gained from DMT will undoubtedly contribute to broader discussions about spirituality, healing, and the nature of reality itself.

NOTE

www.ingramcontent.com/pod-product-compliance
Lightning Source LLC
Chambersburg PA
CBHW070156230526
45471CB00002B/687